FELKENDRAIS METHOD FOR ATHLETES

A Complete Guide For Unraveling Potential And Discovering Fluidity Through Awareness

WALTER ZYAIRE

DISCLAIMER

The information in this book is intended only for general informational purposes; it should not be used in lieu of professional advice or medical care. Since the author is not licensed to practice therapy, the information offered should not be used in place of the expertise, judgment, or guidance of qualified mental health or medical professionals. Readers are encouraged to consult therapists, medical specialists, or other qualified authorities regarding their particular situation and needs. The publisher and author disclaim all liability for any actions or decisions taken by readers based on the information in this book. Results may vary from person to person and this book's approaches, procedures, and strategies may not be suitable in all circumstances. Considering unique situations and consulting a qualified expert are essential when choosing the right course of action. Neither the publisher nor the author recommend or guarantee the efficacy of any therapy or treatment that is indicated in this book. Because the information is based on the author's research and understanding at the time of publishing, it could not reflect the most recent developments or practices in the treatment area. The publisher and the author both disclaim all liability for the accuracy, completeness, or use of the material in this book. Readers bear full responsibility for the decisions and actions they choose in light of the information presented in this book.

TABLE OF CONTENTS

CHAPTER ONE 13

OVERVIEW OF FELDENKRAIS METHOD FOR ATHLETES........................13

THE FELKENDRAIS METHOD'S HISTORY 13

THE FELKENDRAISMETHOD'S BASIS 14

FUNDAMENTALS AND PHILOSOPHIES..14

RECOGNISING MOVEMENT-BASED AWARENESS (ATM)....................15

EXAMINING INTEGRATION OF FUNCTIONS (FI) 16

CHAPTER TWO 17

ADVANTAGES FOR SPORTSMEN 17

INCREASING SELF-AWARENESS...17

INCREASING THE EFFECTIVENESS OF MOVEMENT 17

PREVENTING INJURIES AND PROVIDING REHABILITATION 18

MENTAL SIGHT AND ATTENTION: 19

CHAPTER THREE 21

ATHLETIC MIND-BODY CONNECTION..21

PRACTICING MOVEMENT-BASED MINDFULNESS..............................21

LINKING MOVEMENT AND BREATH 22

THE SIGNIFICANCE OF IMAGINATION AND VISUALISATION 23

DEVELOPING AN UPBEAT ATTITUDE 24

CHAPTER FOUR 25

USING FELKENDRAIS TO SPORTS CONDITIONING...............................25

INCLUDING FELKENDRAIS INTO EXERCISES FOR WARM-UP 25

PARTICULAR METHODS FOR VARIOUS SPORTS 26

TAILORING TRAINING TO SPECIFIC ATHLETES..................................26

EXAMPLES OF SPORTSPEOPLE WHO GAINED FROM 27

CHAPTER FIVE..29

ATHLETIC MIND-BODY CONNECTION...29

INCREASING MOVEMENT-BASED MINDFULNESS 29

LINKING MOVEMENT AND BREATH 29

THE SIGNIFICANCE OF IMAGINATION AND VISUALISATION 30

DEVELOPING AN UPBEAT ATTITUDE 31

CHAPTER SIX...33

TYPICAL MOVEMENT SEQUENCES AND ADJUSTMENTS 33

DETERMINING INADEQUATE MOVEMENT PATTERNS 33

RESOLVING BIOMECHANICAL DISPROPORTIONS............................34

OPTIMAL POSTURE CORRECTION FOR SPORTS PERFORMANCE........35

CHAPTER SEVEN 37

INCLUDING FELKENDRAIS INTO COURSES OF STUDY.........................37

INCLUDING FELKENDRAIS IN FREQUENT EXERCISE PROGRAMMERS 37

WORKING TOGETHER WITH TRAINERS AND COACHES.......................38

DEVELOPING COMPREHENSIVE PROGRAMMES FOR ATHLETE.........38

CHAPTER EIGHT...41

FELKENDRAIS AND RECUPERATED INJURIES 41

FELDENKRAIS-BASED REHAB TECHNIQUES 41

CASE STUDIES FOR THE REHABILITATION OF INJURIES....................42

INCREASING AWARENESS TO PREVENT RECURRENT INJURIES.........43

CHAPTER NINE 45

EXERCISES AND TEACHINGS FOR REAL-WORLD ATHLETES 45

FELKENDRAIS EXAMPLE EXERCISES FOR VARIOUS SPORTS..............45

EXERCISES FOR ATHLETES' SELF-CARE..46

AUDIO-VISUAL MATERIALS FOR ASSISTED LEARNING 47

CHAPTER TEN 49

INCLUDING FELKENDRAIS INTO'S PERFORMANCE IN THE COMPETITION
....49

PREPARING FOR THE COMPETITION 49

METHODS USED IN-GAME/APPLICATION 50

RECUPERATION AFTER COMPETITION 51

CHAPTER ELEVEN 53

BEYOND SPORTS: USING FELKENDRAISM IN EVERYDAY SITUATIONS....53

APPLYING KNOWLEDGE TO ROUTINE TASKS 53

PRESERVING LONG-TERM GAINS 54

FELKENDRA IS FOR GENERAL WELFARE 55

ABOUT THE BOOK

The "Felkendrais Method for Athletes" book is a valuable resource for everyone involved in sports or physical training. This extensive manual, which is intended for athletes of different levels and sports, is based on the Felkendrais Method, which has a long history and origins.

The book gives readers a background on the Felkendrais Method and outlines its guiding principles and philosophy in the introduction. It lays out the goals of the book and highlights how it can benefit a wide range of athletes who want to improve their mental toughness, avoid injuries, and perform better.

The book explores the fundamentals of the Felkendrais Method, such as what Awareness through Movement (ATM) is and how to study Functional Integration (FI). These ideas create the foundation for athletes to become more aware of their bodies and to move more efficiently.

The book delves further into the several advantages that the Felkendrais Method provides for athletes. The benefits of the approach are explained along with how it promotes mental focus and concentration, increases body awareness, increases movement efficiency, and helps prevent and treat injuries. It is a priceless tool for athletes aiming for peak performance and well-being because of these advantages.

Taking a hands-on approach it describes how athletes can incorporate the Felkendrais Method into their training plans. It looks at how to incorporate Felkendrais into warm-up routines, customize sessions for other sports, and provide case studies that highlight the benefits for certain athletes.

The book goes into further detail about the importance of the mind-body link in sports, highlighting the role of breath, the growth of mindfulness in movement, and the influence of imagination and visualization on sports performance.

Typical movement patterns and corrections are discussed, along with methods for incorporating Felkendrais into training regimens. Resolving biomechanical imbalances and improving posture are emphasized as essential elements in improving sports performance.

In addition, the book delves deeper into the topic of injury recovery, explaining rehabilitation techniques and providing case examples that demonstrate how Felkendrais works to prevent repeat injuries by raising awareness.

The ensuing chapters provide useful exercises, teachings, and a comprehensive strategy for incorporating Felkendrais into everyday life—not just as a technique for athletes but also as a means of promoting general well-being. It offers thorough guidance for athletes looking to incorporate Felkendrais into competitive performance, including everything from pre-competition preparation to in-game/application tactics and post-competition rehabilitation.

"Felkendrais Method for Athletes" offers a comprehensive approach to physical and mental well-being, making it an invaluable tool for coaches, athletes, and fitness aficionados alike. This book is a valuable resource for anyone looking to maximize their athletic performance and create a long-lasting bond between the body and mind since it combines theory, practical application, and real-world case studies.

CHAPTER ONE

OVERVIEW OF FELKENDRAIS METHOD FOR ATHLETES

THE FELKENDRAIS METHOD'S HISTORY

Dr. Moshe Feldenkrais created the Felkendrais Method, a comprehensive method for movement and self-awareness that tries to improve both mental and physical health. The methodology emphasizes the complex relationship between body and mind and is based on somatic education and neuroplasticity theories.

Its roots can be found in the wide range of disciplines that Dr. Feldenkrais studied, including psychology, engineering, physics, and martial arts. This multidisciplinary basis established the framework for an approach that promotes self-awareness and enhanced performance.

THE FELKENDRAISMETHOD'S BASIS

The personal journey of Dr. Moshe Feldenkrais, the originator of the Felkendrais Method, serves as the foundation for the method. Felkendra was born in 1904 and experienced physical difficulties as a result of a knee injury. This drove him to investigate different movement modalities to heal. The system was developed in part because of his extensive knowledge of anatomy and biomechanics, as well as his Judo experiences. In the middle of the 20th century, the Felkendrais Method became formally recognized for its unique and unconventional approach to movement education.

FUNDAMENTALS AND PHILOSOPHIES

The underlying assumption of the Felkendrais Method is that the nervous system is inherently capable of self-adaptation and self-reorganization. Dr. Felkendrais developed a method that highlights the brain's capacity to establish new neural connections and patterns throughout life by drawing inspiration from his scientific expertise, including neuroplasticity. According to the approach, people can unleash more potential for effective and graceful functioning by honing their awareness of their movement habits, which will ultimately improve their general well-being.

RECOGNISING MOVEMENT-BASED AWARENESS (ATM)

A fundamental element of the Felkendrais Method is Awareness Through Movement (ATM), which consists of a sequence of guided classes intended to increase self-awareness via movement investigation. The voice instructions in these classes encourage participants to move mindfully and gently while focusing on different body areas. ATM sessions provide a forum for introspection, allowing participants to get a deeper comprehension of their ingrained movement patterns and to build more sophisticated and flexible gaits.

EXAMINING INTEGRATION OF FUNCTIONS (FI)

Another aspect of the Felkendrais Method is called Functional Integration (FI), which entails one-on-one sessions with a practitioner guiding a patient through customized movement explorations using verbal cues and gentle touch. FI sessions, in contrast to ATM, are customized to each person's requirements and experiences to address particular movement problems, reducing discomfort, and improving general functioning. Because Functional Integration is customized, mobility improvement can be approached in a more subtle and focused manner.

The Felkendrais Method is an all-encompassing and cutting-edge strategy for self-awareness and movement education. With a deep historical foundation and guidance from somatic education and neuroplasticity principles, the technique offers a distinctive viewpoint on the relationship between the mind and body.

CHAPTER TWO

ADVANTAGES FOR SPORTSMEN

INCREASING SELF-AWARENESS

Improving one's awareness of one's body is an essential component for athletes looking to maximize their potential. This idea entails becoming more aware of one's body, including how it moves, positions itself, and reacts to outside stimuli. Athletes can develop a closer bond with their bodies by engaging in practices like yoga, Pilates, and particular proprioceptive exercises. This increased awareness helps athletes perform motions more precisely and effectively by enhancing their balance, coordination, and general body control.

INCREASING THE EFFECTIVENESS OF MOVEMENT

Athlete performance is largely determined by their ability to move efficiently, and different training approaches concentrate on improving the biomechanics of particular movements. Through focused exercises and drills, athletes can refine their movement patterns, which can decrease energy waste, improve speed, and boost overall efficiency. This lowers the chance of fatigue-related injuries while simultaneously improving performance. Coaches frequently stress the value of good technique and biomechanics because these skills help players move more efficiently, which improves performance on the pitch or in competition.

PREVENTING INJURIES AND PROVIDING REHABILITATION

The physical demands of their activities often put athletes at risk for injury. Maintaining long-term sporting careers requires training regimens that incorporate measures for preventing injuries. Programs for strength and fitness that target deficiencies, flexibility problems, and muscular imbalances can greatly lower the risk of injuries.

When injuries do happen, recovery becomes crucial. The goal of rehabilitation programs is to regain strength, mobility, and function so that athletes can safely resume their sport with a lower chance of re-injury. Athletes' general well-being and ability to compete are enhanced by comprehensive injury management.

MENTAL SIGHT AND ATTENTION:

In sports, the mental component of performance is frequently just as important as the physical. An athlete's capacity to perform well under duress and make snap decisions can be significantly impacted by mental focus and attention. Improving mental toughness and focus requires the application of strategies like mindfulness meditation, visualization, and cognitive training. Through the mastery of maintaining concentration in the face of distractions and pressure, athletes may consistently perform at their best throughout tournaments. Athletes may face obstacles with a clear and composed head thanks to mental training, which also helps with stress and anxiety management. This leads to an improvement in performance overall.

The advantages for athletes go beyond the realm of the physical and include things like better body awareness, more efficient movements, injury prevention and recovery, and increased mental focus and concentration. In the realm of competitive sports, a comprehensive training program that takes these ideas into account not only improves athletic performance but also promotes long-term physical and mental well-being.

CHAPTER THREE

ATHLETIC MIND-BODY CONNECTION

PRACTICING MOVEMENT-BASED MINDFULNESS

One of the most important aspects of the mind-body connection in sports is mindfulness in movement. It entails practicing presence and awareness during physical activity so that athletes may completely interact with their bodies and environment. Sportsmen can improve their overall performance and lessen the negative effects of distractions by concentrating on the here and now without passing judgment. Practices like yoga, tai chi, or mindful jogging, which teach athletes to observe their body's sensations, movements, and surroundings without reacting, are common ways to cultivate mindfulness in movement. This increased consciousness creates a stronger bond between the body and mind, which enhances the athletic experience and makes it more efficient and harmonious.

LINKING MOVEMENT AND BREATH

Optimizing sports performance fundamentally involves synchronizing breath and movement. In addition to guaranteeing a continuous supply of oxygen to the muscles, conscious breath control also helps control energy levels and improves concentration. To synchronize their breath with different activities, athletes often use specific breathing techniques like diaphragmatic breathing or rhythmic breathing.

In addition to enhancing physical coordination, this link between breath and movement is an effective technique for stress and anxiety management. Athletes can access a natural rhythm that improves their overall performance and helps create a more balanced mind-body connection by intentionally integrating breath into their exercise.

THE SIGNIFICANCE OF IMAGINATION AND VISUALISATION

Imagination and visualization are essential components of the mind-body link in sports. Athletes use mental visualization to see themselves carrying out particular moves, conquering obstacles, or reaching their objectives. This cognitive rehearsal improves confidence, sharpens muscle memory, and improves motor skills. Additionally, visualization stimulates the subconscious, which modifies belief systems and fosters optimism. Athletes prepare their bodies for optimal performance by envisioning successful outcomes in detail, which builds a connection between the mental and physical parts of their athletic endeavors. In the world of sports, the capacity to see and visualize achievement has a substantial positive impact on mental toughness, concentration, and general well-being.

DEVELOPING AN UPBEAT ATTITUDE

One of the main components of the mind-body link in sports is developing an optimistic outlook. Developing optimism, resiliency, and self-belief are all components of a positive mentality and have a direct effect on an athlete's performance. Gratitude exercises, goal-setting, and positive affirmations all aid in the formation of a positive mental attitude. This way of thinking affects an athlete's capacity to overcome obstacles as well as the physiological reactions of the body. Studies show that having a positive outlook can improve physical performance, speed up recuperation, and lower stress levels. Through deliberate cultivation of positivity, athletes establish a balanced connection between their mental and physical states, ultimately realizing their maximum potential and attaining optimal performance in their preferred sport.

CHAPTER FOUR

USING FELKENDRAIS TO SPORTS CONDITIONING

INCLUDING FELKENDRAIS INTO EXERCISES FOR WARM-UP

With its focus on developing better movement patterns and body awareness, Feldenkrais offers a distinctive method for athletic training warm-ups. Incorporating Felkendrais principles into the warm-up helps enhance proprioception and mindfulness, as opposed to concentrating only on traditional stretches or aerobic exercises.

Athletes can create a more conscious connection with their bodies, increasing flexibility and lowering the chance of injury, by moving slowly and deliberately and focusing on their bodily sensations. This integration primes the neuromuscular system for peak performance in addition to readying the body physically for activity.

PARTICULAR METHODS FOR VARIOUS SPORTS

A crucial component of using Felkendrais approaches in athletic training is customizing them to meet the unique requirements of different sports. For instance, Felkendrais training that focuses on fluidity and accuracy in rotating motions may be beneficial to a tennis player since they will improve the agility needed for successful serves and volleys. A long-distance runner, on the other hand, would concentrate on developing effective breathing techniques and maximizing their gait. Because of Felkendra's adaptability, its principles may be tailored to the specific needs of other sports, giving athletes a comprehensive strategy for enhancing the quality of their movements overall.

TAILORING TRAINING TO SPECIFIC ATHLETES

Applying Felkendrais to athletic training requires an understanding of each athlete's uniqueness. Tailoring training sessions to each athlete's unique requirements, strong points, and areas for development guarantees a focused and individualized approach. For example, a sprinter might need to work on explosive movements and fast transitions, whereas a basketball player might benefit from balance and coordination workouts. Through customization of Felkendrais sessions to each athlete's qualities, coaches and practitioners can target particular issues and promote a more thorough development of their physical skills.

EXAMPLES OF SPORTSPEOPLE WHO GAINED FROM FELDENKRAIS

Analyzing case studies yields concrete proof of Felkendrais can's beneficial effects on sports performance. After including Felkendrais into in their training regimes, athletes from a variety of disciplines have claimed increases in their flexibility, coordination, and general body awareness. Targeted Felkendrais sessions, for example, may provide alleviation and a better range of motion for a gymnast who is dealing with chronic joint discomfort.

These case studies demonstrate how Felkendrais to may be tailored to meet the specific demands of each user and highlight its potential as an effective tool for improving sports performance and reducing injuries.

The various advantages of integrating Felkendrais principles into athletic training are illustrated by incorporating them into warm-up routines, using particular approaches for various sports, tailoring sessions to the needs of individual athletes, and reviewing case studies. Athletes can increase their physical skills and develop a better awareness of their bodies by adopting this thoughtful and holistic approach, which will ultimately lead to improved performance and well-being in their respective sports.

CHAPTER FIVE

ATHLETIC MIND-BODY CONNECTION

INCREASING MOVEMENT-BASED MINDFULNESS

One of the most important aspects of the mind-body connection in sports is learning to be conscious when moving. Being mindful entails paying attention to one's thoughts, feelings, and physical sensations while letting go of judgment and living in the present now. Cultivating mindfulness in movement in the context of sports is becoming acutely aware of the movements and reactions of the body while engaging in physical activity. By paying close attention to the feelings associated with each movement, athletes can improve their performance and establish a stronger mental-physical bond.

LINKING MOVEMENT AND BREATH

Another essential component of the mind-body connection in athletics is the integration of breath and movement. The body's conscious and unconscious parts are connected by the breath. The incorporation of appropriate breathing techniques into sports pursuits has the potential to augment physical performance, modulate stress responses, and foster holistic welfare. In addition to maximizing oxygen intake, athletes who time their breathing to match their movements also produce a smooth, flowing motion that enhances their coordination and efficiency.

THE SIGNIFICANCE OF IMAGINATION AND VISUALISATION

In the mind-body link, visualization and imagination are essential components that impact an athlete's physical and mental performance. Visualization is the process of forming clear, vivid mental pictures of actions that will lead to desired results. Athletes can improve muscle memory and boost confidence by frequently visualizing themselves performing a skill or accomplishing a goal. Contrarily, imagination gives players the freedom to consider uncharted territory, which promotes innovation in problem-solving and flexibility in the field. Imagination and visualization both help to develop a resilient and flexible mind, which is necessary in the fast-paced world of sports.

DEVELOPING AN UPBEAT ATTITUDE

One of the most important aspects of the mind-body link in athletics is developing an optimistic outlook. Developing optimism, resiliency, and self-belief are all components of a positive mentality. Positive-thinking athletes are better able to overcome obstacles, bounce back from failures, and stay motivated. An athlete's physical performance can be directly impacted by positive thinking since it lowers stress, improves focus, and fosters general well-being.

It takes deliberate work to establish a positive attitude; this work frequently entails self-talk techniques, mental conditioning, and the creation of a growth-oriented viewpoint that views setbacks as chances for development.

The mind-body link in sports refers to several interrelated ideas that all have a role in an athlete's overall health and performance. Athletes can realize their greatest potential when they cultivate a positive mindset, use their imagination and visualization skills, connect their breath to movement, and develop mindfulness in their movements. By adopting these ideas, players can develop mental toughness, inventiveness, and a comprehensive approach to sports achievement in addition to improving their physical ability.

CHAPTER SIX

TYPICAL MOVEMENT SEQUENCES AND ADJUSTMENTS

DETERMINING INADEQUATE MOVEMENT PATTERNS

Identifying inefficient movement patterns is essential for enhancing sports performance and averting any harm. Seeing asymmetries or abnormalities in a person's movement patterns is essential. This entails examining the way the body moves throughout different workouts or activities and closely monitoring any departures from a biomechanically effective path. Improper alignment, compensatory motions, or inadequate energy transfer are examples of these suboptimal habits.

Furthermore, evaluating movement patterns necessitates comprehending the neuromuscular regulation of distinct muscle segments. To overcome constraints, the body may develop compensatory behaviors as a result of weaknesses or imbalances in specific muscles. To find the underlying source of movement inefficiencies, identifying these compensations frequently entails evaluating the kinetic chain and keeping a sharp eye.

RESOLVING BIOMECHANICAL DISPROPORTIONS

Correcting biomechanical imbalances is crucial for maximizing performance and lowering the risk of injury since they frequently lead to less-than-ideal movement patterns. Several things, including joint constraints, muscular weakness, and tightness, can cause imbalances. To identify particular areas of concern, a comprehensive technique entails doing a full mobility evaluation.

The significance of corrective exercises is crucial in resolving biomechanical abnormalities. The purpose of these exercises is to lengthen tight muscles, strengthen weak ones, and improve joint mobility.

Repetitive functional motions that imitate actions unique to a given activity can be very useful in correcting imbalances and improving overall sports performance. Unilateral exercises also ensure that both sides of the body are equally developed and functional, which helps resolve asymmetries.

Additionally, including mobility drills and flexibility exercises in training regimens helps improve joint range of motion and biomechanics. Regular evaluation and monitoring are essential to determine the efficacy of corrective measures and make required modifications as a person advances through their training.

OPTIMAL POSTURE CORRECTION FOR SPORTS PERFORMANCE

In sports, posture is crucial because it affects power production, movement efficiency, and injury prevention. To correct posture, the body must be positioned to maximize biomechanical function.

This covers posture throughout different tasks, both static and dynamic.

Assessments of static posture can identify abnormalities in the spine, pelvis, and limbs. Typical abnormalities like rounded shoulders or an anterior pelvic tilt might lead to less-than-ideal movement patterns. To treat these problems, specific workouts that strengthen core muscles, realign the spine, and increase general postural awareness must be implemented.

Dynamic posture is equally significant when it is seen in motion. Athletes must stay properly aligned when doing acts unique to their sport. Efficient movement patterns are a result of the kinetic chain being coordinated and each joint operating at its best. Training regimens that include functional exercises and sport-specific drills develop proper posture during dynamic activity.

CHAPTER SEVEN

INCLUDING FELKENDRAIS INTO COURSES OF STUDY

INCLUDING FELKENDRAIS IN FREQUENT EXERCISE PROGRAMMERS

Adding Felkendrais to regular training regimens is a novel way to improve overall athletic performance. Moshe Feldenkrais created the Felkendrais Method, which aims to increase flexibility, body awareness, and movement efficiency.

Enhanced kinesthetic awareness and improved motor abilities can be obtained by athletes by implementing Felkendrais principles into their regular training regimens. To achieve this integration, Felkendrais exercises must be incorporated into warm-ups, cool-downs, and even stand-alone training sessions.

WORKING TOGETHER WITH TRAINERS AND COACHES

Effective integration of Felkendrais into athletic training requires cooperation between coaches and trainers. Felkendra practitioners and sports professionals must effectively communicate to customize the approach to the unique requirements and objectives of the athletes. The needs of the sport can be better understood by coaches, who can then use this knowledge to create Felkendrais workouts that enhance and complement the overall training program. By combining the attentive movement concepts of Feldenkrais with traditional sports training, this partnership promotes a holistic approach.

DEVELOPING COMPREHENSIVE PROGRAMMES FOR ATHLETE DEVELOPMENT

Developing programs for the holistic development of athletes requires a thorough strategy that takes into account the mental, emotional, and physical components of performance. Felkendra can be extremely important in these programs because she brings a mind-body connection that goes beyond traditional training techniques.

Through the use of principles in holistic athlete development, athletes can achieve increased proprioception, better body alignment, and less chance of injury. These programs can be made to incorporate mindfulness exercises in addition to physical activities, which can help athletes become more robust and well-rounded by fostering mental toughness and attention.

Incorporating Felkendrais into regular training regimens offers a novel strategy for athlete development. Working together with trainers and coaches guarantees that the principles are applied in a way that best suits the demands of athletes participating in a variety of sports.

The impact is further enhanced by the development of holistic athlete development programs that address the mental, emotional, and physical aspects of performance. The addition of Felkendra to training regimens is a testament to the way sports science and the quest for peak athletic performance are developing, as interest in its advantages grows.

CHAPTER EIGHT

FELKENDRAIS AND RECUPERATED INJURIES

FELDENKRAIS-BASED REHAB TECHNIQUES

Moshe Feldenkrais created the somatic education technique known as Feldenkrais, which is becoming more and more well-known for its success in helping people recover from injuries. To alleviate physical constraints, the technique focuses on encouraging mindful movement and improving bodily awareness. Felkendrais emphasizes the quality of movement over quantity in rehabilitation, pushing patients to experiment with and improve their movements to restore functional capacities.

Practitioners can support neuromuscular reeducation by using gentle and exploratory activities, which can help people regain balance and a sense of connection with their bodies.

The focus placed by Felkendrais rehabilitation procedures on neuroplasticity—the brain's capacity to reorganize itself in response to experience—is a key component. Practitioners try to stimulate the nervous system by carefully planning movement sequences, which can lead to adaptive changes that can aid in the healing process. This strategy is consistent with the notion that improving coordination, flexibility, and general physical function can be fostered by fine-tuning movement patterns, which in turn can aid in the rehabilitation of injuries.

CASE STUDIES FOR THE REHABILITATION OF INJURIES

Several case studies demonstrate how effective Felkendrais on injury rehabilitation is for a variety of demographics. These studies frequently concentrate on particular injuries, like problems with the musculoskeletal system, neurological disorders, or persistent pain. The exploratory and personalized aspect of Felkendrais sessions, which tailor movements to meet each person's particular needs, is a recurring theme in these situations. These case studies highlight Felkendra's adaptability as an alternative to conventional rehabilitation techniques.

After participating in Felkendrais sessions, people healing from musculoskeletal ailments including sprains, strains, or post-surgical rehabilitation have reported increased functional skills, decreased pain, and a greater range of motion. Positive results have also been observed in neurological diseases like as stroke and traumatic brain injuries, where clients have improved their motor coordination and balance by using the gentle and flexible movements taught in Felkendrais sessions.

INCREASING AWARENESS TO PREVENT RECURRENT INJURIES

Developing an awareness of one's body and movement patterns is a fundamental component of Felkendrais is, which helps to prevent repetitive injuries. A greater awareness of one's body makes one more sensitive to minor indications of strain or imbalance, which enables early intervention and the adjustment of movement patterns. By using a sequence of supervised motions and activities, instructors hope to establish a lasting sense of awareness in their students, enabling them to make deliberate decisions in their everyday lives.

To prevent repetitive injuries, Feldenkrais emphasizes teaching people about their specific movement tendencies and giving them the means to adjust their behavior. In addition to treating current injuries, this proactive strategy seeks to provide the groundwork for long-term well-being. People can create a more resilient and adaptable relationship with their bodies by incorporating awareness into their movement, which lowers their chance of sustaining injuries in the future and increases their overall physical resilience.

CHAPTER NINE

EXERCISES AND TEACHINGS FOR REAL-WORLD ATHLETES

FELKENDRAIS EXAMPLE EXERCISES FOR VARIOUS SPORTS

The Felkendrais Method is a somatic education system that provides athletes with an innovative way to improve their flexibility, body awareness, and overall performance. Customized Felkendrais exercises meet the unique requirements of sportsmen participating in different sports. A light class for runners might concentrate on improving leg quality of movement, with an emphasis on fluidity and effective stride mechanics. Exercises that focus on the fusion of breath and movement can help swimmers become more coordinated and develop more efficient strokes. Felkendrais lessons that focus on balance, agility, and the subtle coordination needed for accurate and powerful shots may be beneficial for tennis players. Athletes can maximize their athletic potential and reach their full movement potential by tailoring Felkendrais workouts to certain sports.

EXERCISES FOR ATHLETES' SELF-CARE

Since athletes frequently have to endure demanding physical conditions, self-care is a crucial part of their training regimen. Self-care techniques extend beyond the traditional definition of rest and recovery to include a comprehensive approach to well-being. Athletes might benefit from incorporating mindfulness practices like deep breathing exercises and meditation to help them manage stress and build mental resilience. Furthermore, self-myofascial release using massage equipment or foam rolling can reduce muscular strain and increase flexibility. Getting enough sleep, eating right, and drinking enough water are essential aspects of self-care that help you perform at your best in sports. Athletes who prioritize self-care not only improve their physical prowess but also develop a balanced, sustainable lifestyle that supports long-term success.

AUDIO-VISUAL MATERIALS FOR ASSISTED LEARNING

Audio and video materials are essential for offering supervised training sessions that improve performance and skill development in the field of athlete development. Athletes can obtain important insights on mental conditioning and attention on the go with the use of audio resources like podcasts or guided meditation sessions. Athletes can watch and imitate proper techniques through visual resources such as instructional videos and virtual coaching platforms, which improves their knowledge and performance of actions. By incorporating these tools into training regimens, athletes can get professional advice from a distance, giving them schedule flexibility. Whether it's correcting techniques for weightlifting or honing a golf swing, audio and visual materials give athletes easily available tools to improve their talents and stay focused on their training goals.

CHAPTER TEN

INCLUDING FELKENDRAIS INTO'S PERFORMANCE IN THE COMPETITION

PREPARING FOR THE COMPETITION

A somatic educational technique called Feldenkrais provides insightful information about how to improve competitive performance in the lead-up to a tournament. The approach places a strong emphasis on better bodily functionality and heightened awareness of movement patterns. Felkendrais an practitioners can concentrate on honing proprioception and kinesthetic awareness during the pre-competition period to help athletes become more attuned to their bodies' subtle cues. This increased awareness can lay the groundwork for successful competitive endeavors by enhancing movement efficiency and lowering the chance of injury.

Pre-competition training with Felkendrais includes a purposeful investigation of movement options. Gentle and mindful exercises are performed by practitioners to enhance muscle function, flexibility, and coordination. Through the integration of these components into their training regimen, athletes can cultivate a deeper bond between their mental and physical selves. This increased connection not only improves performance on the physical level but also fosters a mental state that is beneficial to concentration and focus, which are essential for success in competition.

METHODS USED IN-GAME/APPLICATION

The incorporation of Felkendrais tactics can be very helpful in maximizing an athlete's performance during competition. In this environment, the emphasis on increased awareness and effective movement patterns becomes very pertinent. Principles can help athletes adjust to changing and unforeseen circumstances, enabling them to make more intuitive decisions in a split second.

Felkendrais in-game strategies include the investigation of alternate routes and the constant improvement of movement. Athletes can more skillfully handle the mental and physical demands of competition by implementing these methods. The approach promotes flexibility, enabling players to adjust to the shifting needs of the game with grace and agility. Furthermore, the focus on body awareness and breathing can help with composure under pressure, which is an essential component of winning in competition.

RECUPERATION AFTER COMPETITION

For long-term recuperation and sustained performance, the post-competition phase is essential. Felkendrais addresses the athlete's physical, mental, and emotional well-being to provide a comprehensive approach to post-competition recuperation. To relieve tension that has built up during competition, gentle movements, and guided explorations can be used to encourage relaxation and healing.

Felkendrais post-competition recuperation also incorporates mindfulness and introspection. Athletes are urged to evaluate their performance, acknowledge their successes, and draw lessons from setbacks. This reflective component supports mental development and resilience. Moreover, Felkendrais recovery treatments emphasize alignment optimization and balance restoration to support the body's inherent healing processes.

Incorporating Felkendrais info's competitive performance is a thorough strategy that includes pre-competition planning, in-game tactics, and post-competition recuperation. Through a commitment to the concepts of acute awareness, effective movement, and overall health, athletes can reach their greatest potential and create a long-term blueprint for success in the game.

CHAPTER ELEVEN

BEYOND SPORTS: USING FELKENDRAISM IN EVERYDAY SITUATIONS

APPLYING KNOWLEDGE TO ROUTINE TASKS

Using Felkendrais m in daily life is unique since it emphasizes applying abilities discovered through movement exploration to a variety of daily tasks. Developed by Moshe Feldenkrais, the Felkendrais Method is based on the idea that better awareness and effective movement patterns acquired through certain exercises or courses can transfer into better performance in everyday work. This program goes beyond the field of sports and touches everyday tasks like sitting, walking, and reaching for objects.

People who do Felkendrais become more attentive to their body's feelings and learn how to move more easily and efficiently through the process of somatic learning. Lessons that address the alignment and coordination of the spine, for instance, can help students maintain better posture when doing tasks like standing in line or sitting at a computer. Felkendrais sessions' deliberate and focused movement cultivates a harmonious integration of increased motor function into daily work by acting as a link between athletic talents and the complex demands of daily living.

PRESERVING LONG-TERM GAINS

Felkendrais is a comprehensive method that seeks to provide long-term advantages rather than just a temporary fix for physical pain or a way to improve sports performance. Beyond the time of individual sessions, the method's emphasis on awareness and mindfulness encourages practitioners to incorporate these concepts into their daily lives. Long-term maintenance of the beneficial alterations brought about by Felkendrais depends on this continuity.

Frequent practice develops a more acute awareness of one's body, allowing one to identify and correct habitual movement patterns that may be causing pain or injury. Long-term benefits are more likely as these patterns are gradually replaced with more comfortable and efficient motions. Additionally, the focus on self-awareness and flexibility enables people to respond to the changing requirements of their bodies, fostering long-term well-being outside of the immediate context of athletic endeavors.

FELKENDRA IS FOR GENERAL WELFARE

Even outside of its use in certain sports, the Felkendrais Method has significant effects on general health. This method's emphasis on the mind-body link is consistent with a holistic view of health, which acknowledges the close connection between mental and physical well-being. Through slow, exploratory movements, practitioners develop a sense of awareness and presence in addition to honing their physical skills.

The benefits of the Felkendrais Method for general well-being include reduced stress, enhanced emotional stability, and an increased sensation of relaxation.

People can improve their proprioception, reduce tension, and develop a closer bond with their body by moving deliberately and intently. Beyond the boundaries of physical endeavors, this mind-body harmony enhances the quality of everyday life by promoting a more resilient and balanced state. Essentially, Felkendrais used as a technique to enhance physical abilities as well as cultivate a comprehensive sense of well-being that permeates all aspects of life.